Table of Contents

PREVIEW

Dementia describes a group of symptoms affecting memory, thinking and social abilities severely enough to interfere with your daily life. It isn't a specific disease, but several different diseases may cause dementia.

Though dementia generally involves memory loss, memory loss has different causes. Having memory loss alone doesn't mean you have dementia.

Alzheimer's disease is the most common cause of a progressive dementia in older adults, but there are a number of causes of dementia. Depending on the cause, some dementia symptoms may be reversible.

DEMENTIA DIET RECIPES

BREAKFAST

1. Socca Chickpea Pancakes
Prep Time: 5 Minutes

Cook Time: 10 Minutes

Total Time: 20 minutes

Ingredients

- 2 cups chickpea flour Chickpea flour, or garbanzo bean flour, is often sold with other products by Bob's Red Mill.
- 2 cups water Add almond or nut milk for some of the water for even more nutrients
- 2 tablespoons extra virgin olive oil plus more for the pan
- ¼ teaspoon kosher salt
- ¼ teaspoon black pepper freshly ground
- ½ teaspoon turmeric freshly grated or ground, optional
- essential-recipes-socca-chickpea-flour|brainhealthkitchen.com

Instructions

1. Whisk all the ingredients together in a medium bowl. Set batter aside to rest for 10 minutes.

2. Warm 1 teaspoon olive oil in a a 6-inch nonstick skillet over medium heat. Pour in ⅓ cup socca batter and swirl to create an even pancake.

3. After about 2 minutes, air bubbles will appear on the surface of the socca. Use a spatula to release its edges from the pan, then carefully lift and turn over. (Be gentle! Socca are delicate and can easily tear, but they still taste delicious.) Cook on the other side for about 2 minutes, or until it is crispy and starting to brown.

4. Place finished socca on a plate. Eat as is, or topped with whatever you like. Pictured here: hummus, shredded cabbage, cilantro and a sprinkling of Parmesan cheese.

2. Cranberry Chutney

Servings: 2

Ingredients

- 3 cups fresh cranberries
- ½ cup water
- 3 tablespoons date syrup or honey
- 1 teaspoon small jalapeno chile seeds removed, finely diced + 1 to sprinkle on top
- ½ teaspoon ground coriander
- ½ teaspoon ground turmeric
- ¼ teaspoon kosher salt

Instructions

1. Combine the cranberries, water, date syrup, chiles, coriander, turmeric, and salt in a medium saucepan and bring to a boil over medium-high heat. When the cranberries start to pop, reduce the heat to a gentle simmer. Cook, stirring often, until the sauce coats the back of a spoon, 15 to 20 minutes. Sprinkle with more jalapeño before serving.

3. Chai-Spiced Cranberry Apple Compote

Prep Time: 20 Minutes

Cook Time: 35 Minutes

Total Time: 55 minutes

Servings: 3

Ingredients

- 1 cup water
- 1 chai tea bag
- 3 cups fresh cranberries
- 1 cups large tart apple such as a Granny Smith or Honeycrisp, ½-inch dice (about 1½| TK g)
- 2 tablespoons date syrup or honey
- ½ teaspoon ground cardamom
- ¼ teaspoon kosher salt
- ¼ teaspoon reshly ground black pepper
- ¼ cup candied ginger finely diced + more to sprinkle on top.

Instructions

1. Bring the water to a boil in a medium saucepan, add the tea bag, and turn off the heat. Steep for 5 minutes and discard (or reuse) the tea bag. Add the cranberries, apple, date syrup, cardamom, salt, and freshly ground black pepper to the tea and bring to a boil. When the cranberries start to pop, reduce the heat to a gentle simmer. Cook, stirring often, until the

sauce coats the back of a spoon, 15 to 20 minutes. Stir in the candied ginger and sprinkle a few teaspoons on top.

4. Walnut "Parm" with Zucchini Noodles

Prep Time: 10 minutes

Cook Time: 15 minutes

Total Time: 25 minutes

Servings: 4

Ingredients

- For the Walnut "Parm"
- 1 cup raw walnuts
- ¼ cup nutritional yeast
- 2 tablespoons white miso paste
- 1 small garlic clove
- 1 teaspoon smoked salt such as Maldon
- For the Zucchini Noodles
- 2 medium zucchini spiralized into spaghetti-sized noodles, and cut into 6-inch lengths
- 1 tablespoon extra virgin olive oil
- ¼ teaspoon kosher salt

Instructions

Make the Walnut "Parm"

1. Combine all the ingredients in the bowl of a food processor or blender. Pulse until the mixture forms small, uniform crumbles, like wet sand or coarsely grated Parmesan cheese.

2. To Store: Leftover Walnut Parm keeps in an airtight container in the refrigerator for up to one week.

Cook the Zucchini Noodles

1. Heat half the oil in a large skillet over low-medium heat. When it starts to shimmer, add half the zucchini noodles and a pinch of the salt. Cook, tossing often with tongs, until they soften and begin to brown. Transfer to a large shallow bowl. Repeat with the remaining oil and noodles, seasoning with salt as you go.

To Finish

1. Top the zucchini with enough Walnut Parm to coat, about ½ cup. Toss well and add freshly ground pepper to taste. Serve warm or at room temperature.

5. Crispy Cauliflower Tacos with a Creamy Red Pepper Sauce

Prep Time: 25 minutes

Cook Time: 30 minutes

Total Time: 55 minutes

Servings: 4

Ingredients

- 1 small head of cauliflower about 1½ pounds
- 2 teaspoons chili powder
- ½ teaspoon kosher salt
- 1 tablespoon avocado or extra virgin olive oil
- ¼ cup water
- For the Tacos
- ½ cup Creamy Red Pepper Sauce recipe follows
- 4 Corn tortillas warmed
- 1 cup sugar snap peas sliced thin on the bias
- Cilantro leaves for serving
- Crumbled feta cheese for serving
- ¼ cup pickled jalapeño peppers
- 1 lime cut into 4 wedges

Instructions

1. Wash and trim the cauliflower, removing any outer leaves. Using a knife, separate the head in half from the top to the stem. Slice into 3-by3-inch pieces, each about ½-inch thick. (Slicing the cauliflower creates a

flat surface to enable a crispy exterior, and keep them from falling out of your taco. It's fine to just break into florets if you prefer.) Toss in a bowl with the chili powder and salt.

2. To cook the cauliflower, heat a large nonstick skillet (that has a tight-fitting lid) over medium heat. Add the oil, and when it starts to shimmer add the cauliflower pieces, separating them so they do not touch. Once they become brown and crispy on one side, after about 3 minutes, flip them over. Cook until brown and crispy, then carefully pour the water into the skillet and cover. Remove from the heat and let the cauliflower steam in the pan for 1 to 2 minutes, or until easily pierced with a knife.

3. To build your tacos, divide the red pepper sauce, cauliflower, sugar snaps, and jalapenos between the tortillas. Top with cilantro, feta, and a couple pickled jalapeños. Serve each plate with a lime wedge.

6. Citrusy Cod Packets with Zucchini and Quinoa

Prep Time: 10 minutes

Cook Time: 15 minutes

Total Time: 25 minutes

Servings: 4

Ingredients

- 4 4-ounce pieces boneless, skin-on cod filets about 1-inch thick
- ½ cup fresh orange juice plus 2 tablespoons zest
- ⅓ cup fresh lemon juice plus 2 tablespoons zest
- 1 teaspoon kosher salt divided, plus more to taste
- 1 ¾ cups water
- 1 cup quinoa rinsed
- 1 medium zucchini spiralized, about 3 cups
- 3 tablespoons extra virgin olive oil plus more for coating the paper
- 2 medium garlic cloves thinly sliced
- ¼ teaspoon freshly ground black pepper
- 2 blood oranges very thinly sliced into half-moons
- Flaky salt to finish
- Cilantro leaves optional

Instructions

1. Preheat your oven to 400°F.

2. Place the cod in a 1-quart-size rimmed baking dish and pour the juices over them. Flip the fish over a few times so that the pieces are coated with the marinade, then place skin-side down. Sprinkle with ½ teaspoon of the salt, cover, and place in the fridge for at least 20 minutes and up to 1 hour.

3. While the cod marinates, cook the quinoa. Combine the water and quinoa in a medium saucepan with a tight-fitting lid and bring to a boil. Reduce the heat to a low simmer and cook for 15 minutes. Remove the pot from the heat, covered, and let it sit for 10 more minutes. Fluff with a fork when ready to use.

4. Meanwhile, place the zucchini in a medium bowl with the orange and lemon zests, oil, garlic, pepper, and the remaining ½ teaspoon salt. Toss well to coat and set aside.

5. To assemble the packets, lay out four 10-by-14-inch pieces of parchment paper. Fold each sheet in half, forming a 7-by-10-inch rectangle. Use scissors to cut out a half-moon as big as the paper allows. Unfold the half moon of paper into a circle. Brush one half with olive oil, and divide the quinoa, vegetables, and fish pieces (skin-side down) between the four oiled halves. Top each piece of cod with 3 to 4 blood orange slices. Drizzle a few spoonfuls of marinade over the fish.

6. To seal the packets, fold the top half of parchment over the fish and align the edges. Starting at one corner, fold over about ½-inch of the edge 3 times,

pressing down to make a crisp crease after each fold. Continue to work your way around the edge of the packet, making overlapping, pleat-like folds, always pressing firmly and creasing the edge so the folds hold. When you get to the end of the paper, twist it into a tail to prevent the liquid from seeping out. If necessary, make a second fold wherever there doesn't appear to be a tight seal. When finished, your packet will look like a large calzone.

7. Place the packets on a rimmed baking sheet. Bake for 15 minutes. The paper will darken and puff up as the packet fills with steam. Cooking time will depend on the thickness of your fish; allow a few more minutes if your filets are more than 1-inch thick.

8. To serve, transfer the packets to a plate. Using scissors or a sharp knife, slit open the lids of the packets and fold the paper back. Sprinkle with flaky salt and top with cilantro leaves, if using.

7. One-Skillet Huevos

Prep Time: 10 minutes

Cook Time: 10 minutes

Total Time: 20 minutes

Servings: 4

Ingredients

- 1 15-ounce can black beans rinsed
- 1 cup jarred salsa made from red or green chiles (or a mix), mild, medium or hot
- 1 cup nut milk unsweetened and unflavored (such as almond, cashew, macadamia, pecan, or other)
- ½ teaspoon kosher salt
- 4 to 6 large eggs
- 1 avocado sliced
- 1 scallion both white and green parts finely chopped (optional)
- Corn tortillas warmed

Instructions

1. Combine the beans, salsa, nut milk, and salt in a large skillet. Bring to a gentle simmer over medium heat. Use a spoon to make a well in the sauce and crack an egg into it. Repeat with as many eggs as you want to cook and that your skillet allows.

2. Cover tightly and adjust the heat so that the sauce is gently bubbling at a low simmer. Cook for 5 to 8 minutes, depending on how you like your eggs: about 7 minutes for a jammy yolk or longer for a fully cooked one.

3. To serve, scoop out some of the sauce and an egg or two into each bowl. Top with avocado slices and scatter with scallions, if using. Serve with warm tortillas on the side.

8. White Chicken Chili with Hatch Chiles and Black Beans

Prep Time: 10 minutes

Cook Time: 30 minutes

Total Time: 40 minutes

Servings: 4

Ingredients

- Warmed corn tortillas for serving
- 1 tablespoon avocado or extra virgin olive oil
- 1 large yellow onion thinly sliced (about 2 cups)
- 1 teaspoon kosher salt plus more for seasoning the chicken and to taste
- 2 large garlic cloves roughly chopped, (about 1 tablespoon total)
- 2 cups unsweetened almond milk
- 1 cup Hatch chiles roasted, seeded and diced (frozen and defrosted, or from 2 4-ounce cans)
- 1 teaspoon ground cumin
- 1 teaspoon dried oregano
- 1 15-ounce can black beans rinsed
- 1 ½ pounds boneless skinless chicken breasts
- ¼ teaspoon freshly ground black pepper plus more to taste
- 1 handful cilantro leaves and stems roughly chopped
- 1 avocado diced (optional)
- 4 tablespoons cheddar cheese grated (optional)

- 4 tablespoons pickled red onions optional
- 1 cup cooked brown black, or white rice (optional)
- white chicken chili

Instructions

1. Warm the oil in a heavy pot (that has a tight-fitting lid) over medium heat. Add the onions, sprinkle with a ¼ teaspoon of the salt, and cook, stirring occasionally, until soft and starting to brown, about 10 minutes. Reduce the heat to low and add the garlic. Cook for another minute, or until fragrant, being careful not to let it burn.
2. Add the almond milk, chiles, cumin, oregano, black beans, and another teaspoon of the salt to the pot. Bring to a simmer, then reduce the heat until gently bubbling.

3. Season the chicken breasts by sprinkling both sides with the rest of the salt (¼ teaspoon) and the black pepper. Place the chicken breasts gently into the liquid, cover the pot, and cook until you can easily pull the chicken apart with two forks, about 12 minutes.

4. Transfer the chicken to a bowl and set it aside until cool enough to handle, then shred it using two forks. Add the chicken and any juices back into the chili. Simmer until the chili is gently bubbling again. Add salt and freshly ground pepper to taste.

5. To serve, divide evenly between 4 bowls and top with the chili, cilantro, and avocado, pickled onions and cheese (if using) with the tortillas on the side. If you're serving with rice, place in the bowls before topping with chili.

6. To Store: The soup will keep in an airtight container for up to 3 days in the fridge or 3 months in the freezer.

9. Brown Rice Pudding with Roasted Oranges and Chocolate

Prep Time: 10 minutes
Cook Time: 1 hour
Total Time: 1 hour 10 minutes
Servings: 6

Ingredients

- 3 small oranges
- 4 ½ cups unsweetened almond milk
- 1 cup short-grain brown rice rinsed
- ¼ teaspoon cardamom
- ½ teaspoon kosher salt
- 2 tablespoons raw honey
- 1 teaspoon vanilla extract
- ½ teaspoon orange blossom extract optional
- 2 ounces dark chocolate (65-80% cacao) coarsely chopped, or ¼ cup dark chocolate chips
- Flaky salt for serving

Instructions

1. Preheat your oven to 400°F. Scrub the oranges well and wrap them in foil. Roast in the oven for 45 minutes, or until soft and slightly collapsed.

2. Bring the almond milk to a simmer in a medium pot, being careful not to let it boil over. Add the rice, salt,

and cardamom. Simmer uncovered, stirring occasionally, for about 30 minutes or until the rice is tender and there is very little liquid left in the bottom of the pan. Cover with a tight-fitting lid and set the pan away from the heat to steam for 10 minutes.

3. Stir the honey, vanilla extract, and orange blossom water (if using) into the rice pudding.

4. When the roasted oranges are cool enough to handle, cut them in half, pick out any seeds, and scoop out the fruit, pith and all. Set the orange peel "cups" aside to stuff later. Coarsely chop the fruit, and fold it into the pudding. Put aside a few teaspoons of chocolate to sprinkle on each serving, and stir the rest into the pudding.

5. To serve, fill each hollowed out orange half with a generous half cup of rice pudding and sprinkle with the rest of the chocolate and a few pinches of flaky salt. Serve warm or at room temperature.

10. Cinnamon-Spiced Farro Breakfast Bowl with Hazelnuts, Berries, and Honey

Prep Time: 10 minutes

Cook Time: 35 minutes

Total Time: 45 minutes

Servings: 4

Ingredients

- 3 cups water
- 1 cup semi-pearled farro rinsed
- ¼ teaspoon kosher salt
- 1 cup unsweetened almond milk warmed
- 1 teaspoon ground cinnamon
- 1 cup toasted hazelnuts skinned and chopped (see note)
- teaspoon raw honey for drizzling (no more than 1 per serving)
- 2 cups berries fresh or frozen and defrosted
- ¼ cup pumpkin seeds raw or toasted, salted or unsalted, optional
- Cinnamon-Spiced Farro

Instructions

1. Combine the water and farro in a medium saucepan with 3 cups of water.

2. Bring to a boil, then reduce to a simmer and cook over low heat for 25 to 35 minutes, adding the salt in the last 5 minutes of cooking. The farro is done when it is soft and chewy but the grains are still intact.

3. Drain, stir in the cinnamon, and spoon into 4 bowls. Top each bowl with the almond milk, berries, toasted hazelnuts, a drizzle of honey, and pumpkin seeds (if using), dividing evenly.

11. Roasted Caprese with Shrimp, Avocado, and Feta

Prep Time: 10 minutes

Cook Time: 30 minutes

Total Time: 40 minutes

Servings

Ingredients

- 4 roma or plum tomatoes halved lengthwise, seeds scooped out with a sharp spoon
- 1 tablespoon extra virgin olive oil plus more for drizzling
- 1 tablespoon balsamic vinegar
- ¼ teaspoon kosher salt plus more for seasoning
- 8 medium shrimp shelled and deveined
- ½ cup feta roughly chopped
- 1 avocado peeled and cut into ¼-inch slices
- 1 handful fresh basil leaves enough for about 2 for each tomato piece
- freshly ground black pepper to taste

Instructions

1. Preheat your oven to 375°F. Line a rimmed baking sheet with parchment paper.

2. Place the tomato halves on the baking sheet cut-side up. Drizzle the oil and vinegar evenly over the tomatoes and sprinkle with the salt. Bake for 20 minutes, or until the tomatoes are soft and starting to brown on the edges. Add the shrimp to the baking sheet nestled amongst the tomatoes and drizzle with olive oil. Bake for another 10 minutes.

3. To serve, divide the tomatoes evenly between 4 plates. Top each tomato with a shrimp, a few slices of avocado, feta, and basil. Drizzle with olive oil and sprinkle with more salt and freshly ground black pepper. Serve warm or at room temperature.

12. Roasted Brussels Sprouts, Apple, and Greens Salad

12.Delicious Food

Prep Time: 25 minutes
Cook Time: 45 minutes
Total Time: 1 hour 5 minutes
Servings: 2

Ingredients

- 5 tablespoons extra virgin olive oil
- 2 tablespoons pure maple syrup
- 2 tablespoons balsamic vinegar
- 1 tablespoon low sodium soy sauce or tamari
- 1 clove mediumgarlic minced
- 2 cups Brussels sprouts quartered
- ¼ teaspoon kosher salt
- 6 cups salad greens
- 1 large apple core removed, chopped into ½-inch cubes
- ½ cup walnut halves or pieces
- ¼ cup dried currants
- Flaky sea salt to garnish
- Brussels sprouts, apple and greens salad

Instructions

1. Combine ¼ cup of the oil, the maple syrup, soy sauce, and garlic in a blender. Blend until smooth; set aside.
2. Preheat your oven to 375°F. Toss the Brussels sprouts on a rimmed baking sheet with the remaining tablespoon of oil and the salt. Spread them out so they are all in a single

layer. Roast for 20 minutes, or until the edges are crispy and brown. Set aside to cool.

3. Place the greens in a salad bowl and toss with the cooled Brussels sprouts and 2 tablespoons of the dressing. Toss to combine, then top with the diced apple, walnuts, and currants. Drizzle another 2 tablespoons of dressing and toss well. Sprinkle with flaky sea salt and serve immediately.

13. Garlicky Mushroom and Swiss Chard Manicotti

Servings: 4

Ingredients

For the marinara:

- ¼ cup extra virgin olive oil
- 2 28-ounce can crushed tomatoes
- 3 small garlic cloves minced
- ½ teaspoon kosher salt
- ½ teaspoon dried oregano
- 6 fresh basil leaves torn

For the Socca (chickpea crepes):

- 1 cups water
- 1 large egg
- 1 ¾ cups chickpea flour
- 1 tablespoon extra virgin olive oil plus more for cooking the socca
- 1/4 teaspoon kosher salt
- 2 tablespoons Parmesan cheese freshly grated

For the Filling:

- 4 tablespoons extra virgin olive oil
- 1 pound small mushrooms, such as cremini or white button sliced ¼-inch thick, about 4 cups
- ¾ teaspoon kosher salt
- 3 small garlic cloves minced
- 1 bunch Swiss chard (about ¾ lb.) stems sliced ¼-inch thick, leaves slices ½-inch thick

- ⅛ teaspoon red pepper flakes
- 2 cups store-bought cashew or almond ricotta
- To Top:
- ¼ cup freshly grated Parmesan cheese optional
- Handful fresh basil leaves torn
- Manicotti healthy ingredients

Instructions

1. Make the Marinara: Heat the oil in a large pot over medium heat. When it starts to shimmer, add the crushed tomatoes and garlic. Stir constantly for 2 minutes. Add the oregano and bring to a boil over high heat, then reduce to a gentle simmer. Place a lid ajar on the pot and continue to cook, stirring every 15 minutes, until the sauce is smooth, about 1 hour. Add the torn basil leaves. Taste; add more salt if you like.

2. While the sauce simmers, make the Socca. Using a blender or a large bowl and whisk, combine the water, egg, chickpea flour, oil, and salt until smooth. Stir in the grated Parmesan. Set aside for about 10 minutes to allow the batter to thicken.

3. Heat a 9-inch nonstick skillet over medium-low heat. Add a few drops of oil and ⅓ cup of the batter. Swirl the pan so that the socca is almost as large as the pan. After about 2 minutes, the socca should be set in the middle and crispy at the edges. Carefully slip a flexible spatula under one side of the socca and loosen it from the pan. Slide it onto a flat surface, such as your countertop or a cutting board. If the socca tears a little, you can still use it. Repeat until you have about about 10 socca.

4. Make the filling: Preheat your oven to 400°F. Heat one tablespoon of the oil in a large skillet over medium heat. When it starts to shimmer, add half the mushrooms and a pinch of salt. Spread the

mushrooms out so they are mostly in a single layer, and cook, stirring occasionally, until soft and brown on the edges, about 5 minutes. Transfer the mushrooms to a medium bowl. Repeat with the rest of the mushrooms.

5. Using the same skillet, add another tablespoon of olive oil. Add the chard stems, sprinkle with a pinch of salt, and sauté until soft, about 4 minutes. Add the garlic and cook over low heat, stirring continuously for 1 minute. Add the greens and cook until soft, about 5 minutes. Transfer to the bowl with the mushrooms.

6. Use a fork to break up the ricotta and season it with the red pepper flakes and ¼ teaspoon of salt. Gently fold in the chard and mushrooms until combined.

7. To assemble the manicotti: Pour two cups of marinara sauce on the bottom of a ceramic or glass 9-by-13-inch baking dish. Place a socca on a cutting board and spoon ¼ cup of the filling onto one end. Roll up like a cigar and place seam side down on the baking dish. Repeat until all the manicotti have been made. Arrange the manicotti so there is a tiny bit of space between each and pour 2 more cups of sauce on top. Smooth over the top, cover with foil, and bake for 45 minutes, until the manicotti are brown around the edges and the filling is bubbling and spilling out the ends.

8. Let rest for about 15 minutes. Just before serving, top with fresh basil leaves and a sprinkling of Parmesan cheese, if using.

14. Kale Salad with Persimmons and Spiced Walnuts

Servings:

Ingredients

- 2 tablespoons extra virgin olive oil plus 1 teaspoon for the nuts
- 1 tablespoon freshly squeezed orange or lemon juice
- 1 small garlic clove minced
- ¾ teaspoon kosher salt plus more to taste
- 1 cups bunch lacinato kale leaves torn into bite-sized pieces (about 4total), discard stems or reserve for another use, also known as Tuscan or dinosaur
- 1 cup raw walnut halves or pieces
- 1 teaspoon coconut palm sugar
- ¼ teaspoon ground cumin
- ¼ teaspoon ground cinnamon
- ¼ teaspoon cayenne pepper or chili powder
- ½ small head radicchio sliced ¼-inch thick
- 2 ripe persimmons cored and sliced into ⅛-inch thick rounds, preferably Fuyu
- freshly ground black pepper to taste

Instructions

1. Preheat your oven to 350°F.

2. In a medium salad bowl, whisk 2 tablespoons of the oil, the orange or lemon juice, garlic, and ½ teaspoon salt.

3. Add the kale and radicchio and toss well to coat. Use your hands to ensure all the greens are coated evenly with the dressing. Set aside at room temperature while you make the rest of the salad, at least 20 minutes.

4. Place the walnuts on a small baking sheet. Toast for 5 to 7 minutes, until fragrant and golden brown. Meanwhile, stir together the sugar, cumin, cinnamon, cayenne, and ¼ teaspoon salt in a small bowl; set aside.

5. Heat the remaining teaspoon of oil in large skillet over low heat. Add the toasted walnuts and toss to coat. Remove from the heat and stir in the spices until the walnuts are coated evenly.

6. Add the radicchio to the kale and toss to combine. Top the greens with the persimmons, the spiced walnuts, and any oil from the skillet. Toss until the persimmons are also coated with the dressing. Finish the salad with a pinch more salt and freshly ground black pepper, if you like. Serve immediately.

15. Spiced Nuts with Turmeric and Garam Masala

Servings: 3 cup

Ingredients

- 3 cups mixed unsalted raw nuts (I like equal parts cashews walnuts, and almonds)
- 3 tablespoons avocado or extra virgin olive oil
- 2 teaspoons garam masala see note below
- 1 teaspoon kosher salt
- 1 teaspoon ground chile powder
- 1 teaspoon coconut palm sugar
- 1 teaspoon ground turmeric
- 1 tablespoon chickpea flour

Instructions

1. Preheat your oven to 350°F. Line a rimmed baking sheet with parchment paper; set aside.

2. Combine the nuts and oil in a large mixing bowl and toss until evenly coated. Add the remaining ingredients and toss well so that each nut is evenly coated. Transfer to the prepared baking sheet and smooth into an even layer.

3. Bake until the nuts are fragrant and lightly toasted, about 30 minutes. Check the nuts after 15 minutes, give them a toss, and assess how fast they are cooking. If your oven runs hot, they may be done.

4. Serve warm, or cool completely and save in an airtight container for up to 2 weeks.

16. Apple Tahini Tart with a Maple Oat Crust

Servings: 1

Ingredients

Maple Oat Crust

- 1½ cups old-fashioned rolled oats
- ½ cup almond flour
- ¼ cup extra virgin olive oil
- ¼ cup pure maple syrup
- ¼ teaspoon kosher salt
- 1 large Medjool date, pitted

Tahini Cashew Cream

- 1½ cups raw, unsalted cashews soaked in water for at least 2 hours
- 2 tablespoons pure maple syrup
- 1 tablespoon tahini
- ½ teaspoon kosher salt
- 1¼ cups cold water

For the apples

- 2 large apples such as Gala or Pink Lady, halved, cored and cut into ⅛-inch slices
- ¾ teaspoon cinnamon
- ¾ teaspoon coconut palm sugar

Maple Tahini Drizzle

- 1 tablespoon tahini
- 1 tablespoon pure maple syrup
- 1 tablespoon water

Sesame Seed Topping, optional

- 1 teaspoon white sesame seeds
- ½ teaspoon black sesame seeds

Instruction

Make the Maple Oat Crust:

1. Preheat your oven to 350°F. Place the ingredients for the crust in the bowl of a food processor and pulse until evenly combined.
2. Pour the tart dough onto a 9-inch tart pan with a removable bottom. Cover the dough with wax or parchment paper and, using your hands, press in an even layer all over the bottom and sides of the pan. Use the flat bottom of a glass or a measuring cup to press the crust flat and even. Prick all over with a fork and place on a rimmed baking sheet.
3. Bake the crust for 15 minutes, or until it is set in the middle and light brown. Set aside and let it cool.

While the crust cools, Make the Tahini Cashew Cream

1. Drain the soaked cashews and place them in a blender with the maple syrup, tahini, and salt. Add half the water and turn the blender on medium to combine. Turn it up to high and blend until it looks like whipped cream, adding water by the spoonful until the consistency is just right. Measure out 2 cups for the tart, and store any extra in the refrigerator for up to 5 days.

Assemble the Tart:

1. Pour the cashew cream onto the center of the baked tart shell and smooth it over the surface using a spatula or a spoon. Arrange the apple slices in a concentric circle starting at the outside of the tart and

working to the center. Press the slices gently into the cream. Stir the cinnamon and coconut palm sugar together in a small bowl and sprinkle evenly on the surface of the apples. Return the tart to the oven and bake for 35 to 40 minutes, until the edges of the apples are browned and the crust is golden brown. Let the tart cool for about 30 minutes.

While the tart cools, make the Maple Tahini Drizzle:

2. In a small bowl, stir together the tahini, maple syrup and just enough water to form a pourable glaze, starting with one teaspoon water and adding more if needed. Drizzle in a concentric circle over the surface of the cooled tart, then sprinkle the sesame seeds overtop, if using.
3. To serve, carefully lift the bottom of the tart pan away from its fluted side. Cut into wedges and serve.

17. Portobello Bacon

Prep Time: 10 minutes
Cook Time: 30 minutes
Total Time: 40 minutes
Servings: 4

Ingredients
- 4 cups portobello mushrooms stems removed, caps cut into ½-inch slices
- 2 teaspoons Liquid Smoke
- 4 teaspoons low sodium soy sauce
- 1 teaspoon smoked paprika
- 2 teaspoons maple syrup
- 2 teaspoons Worcestershire sauce
- 2 Tbsp. olive oil
- ½ teaspoon coarse sea salt
- freshly ground pepper to taste

Instructions
1. Preheat the oven to 350°F. Line a rimmed baking sheet with parchment paper or a silicone mat.

2. In a large bowl, whisk together the Liquid Smoke, soy sauce, smoked paprika, maple syrup, Worcestershire sauce, olive oil, salt and pepper.Add the mushrooms and toss gently until all are evenly coated. Marinate for 15 minutes.

3. Pour the mushrooms onto the baking sheet and separate so none are touching. Bake for 30 minutes, flipping after 15, until crispy.

18. Mixed Berry Polenta Crisp

Prep Time: 10 minutes

Cook Time: 40 minutes

Total Time: 50 minutes

Servings: 8

Ingredients

For the berries:

- 8 cups berries blackberries, blueberries, raspberries, or a mix, fresh or frozenno
- 2 oranges zested and juiced
- ½ teaspoon koshersalt

For the crisp topping:

- 4 tablespoons butter preferably grass-fed
- 3 tablespoons extra virgin olive oil
- 1 cup almond flour
- ½ cup quick-cooking polenta also called instant polenta
- ¼ cup coconut palm sugar
- 1 egg
- ½ tsp baking powder
- ½ tsp kosher salt

Instructions

1. Preheat the oven to 375°F.

2. Clean and sort the berries, removing leaves and stems.

3. Place the berries in a 11- by 7-inch ceramic or glass pan. Add orange zest, orange juice, and a pinch of salt. Toss gently so that all the berries are coated.

4. Cut the butter into small cubes and place in a food processor. Add almond flour, polenta, sugar, egg, baking powder, and salt. Pulse 10 times or until a crumbly dough forms. (Or, place all the ingredients in a mixing bowl and crumble them together with your hands.)

5. Crumble the topping over the berries. Place the baking dish on a baking sheet lined with parchment paper for easier clean-up. Bake until the crisp is lightly browned and the filling is bubbling, 30 to 40 minutes. Cool for about 30 minutes before serving to allow the juices to set up and thicken.

19. Farmers Market Veggie Tagine

Prep Time: 30 minutes

Cook Time: 45 minutes

Total Time: 1 hour 15 minutes

Servings: 4

Ingredients

- 1 tsp ground cumin
- 1 tsp ground coriander
- 1/2 tsp cinnamon
- 1/2 tsp red pepper flakes
- 1 tbsp extra virgin olive oil
- 1 yellow onion chopped into 1-inch pieces
- 1/2 tsp coarse salt plus more to taste
- 2 garlic cloves minced
- 1 tsp grated fresh ginger
- 1/2 cup preserved lemon rinsed and cut into slivers
- 1/2 cups vegetable broth
- 8 dried figs diced
- 2 medium sweet potatoes cut into 1-inch pieces
- 4 medium carrots purple and red, cut into 1-inch pieces
- 3 small green zucchini cut into 1-inch pieces
- 1/2 cups cooked chickpeas drained and rinsed
- 2 tbsp fresh lemon juice
- freshly ground black pepper
- 1/2 cup fresh mint choppped

- 1/4 cup sliced almonds toasted
- Homemade Harissa for serving*
- veggie tagine

Instructions

1. In a small bowl, mix together the cumin, coriander, cinnamon, and red pepper flakes. Set aside.
2. Heat the olive oil in a large pot or Dutch oven over medium heat. Add the onion and the salt and cook until soft, about 5 minutes.
3. Reduce the heat to low and stir in the garlic, ginger, preserved lemon, and dried spices. Add the broth, figs, vegetables, and chickpeas. Bring to a gentle boil, then reduce the heat to low and simmer and cook, covered, for 20 minutes.
4. Cook uncovered for about 8 to 10 minutes, stirring occasionally. Once the stew has thickened and the vegetables are al dente, remove from the heat. Add lemon juice and season with salt and freshly ground pepper.
5. Top with mint and almonds just before serving. Serve with Cauliflower Couscous and Homemade Harissa.

20. Summer Vegetable Tian

Prep Time: 30 minutes
Cook Time: 1 hour 10 minutes
Total Time: 1 hour 40 minutes
Servings: 4

Ingredients

- 1/3 cup extra virgin olive oil
- 3 large garlic cloves thinly sliced
- 2-3 medium tomatoes
- 1 medium zucchini
- 1 medium yellow squash
- 1-2 sweet potatoes scrubbed
- 1-2 large red onion
- coarse sea salt about 1 tsp
- Handful of fresh thyme
- summer vegetable tian

Instructions

1. Preheat the oven to 400°F. Rub a 9-inch round baking dish (such as a pie plate) with the cut side of a clove of garlic.

2. Using a mandoline or a sharp knife, slice the vegetables no more than ¼-inch thick. Ideally, all the vegetable slices should be about the same size.

3. Pour half the olive oil into the baking dish. Arrange the vegetable slices in the dish in a

circular pattern, alternating evenly between the tomato, zucchini, sweet potato and onion. Fill the center of the dish with a smaller circle of vegetables. Sprinkle the vegetables liberally with the salt. Tuck the garlic slices between the vegetables evenly throughout the dish.

4. Strip most of the thyme of its leaves, leaving a few intact sprigs for garnish. Drizzle the rest of the olive oil over the top and sprinkle with fresh thyme leaves. Add an additional sprinkle of salt.

5. Bake for 70 to 90 minutes, or until the vegetables are tender. Top with thyme sprigs and cut into triangular pieces. Serve hot or warm.

DINNER

21. Whole Grain Penne with Creamy Squash and Sesame

Servings: 4

Ingredients

- 6 cups cubed butternut squash or pumpkin (from 1 large or 2 small squash, about 3 lbs. total), peeled and divided
- 3 tablespoons extra virgin olive oil
- ¼ cup sesame seeds I like to use equal parts white and black.
- 2 tablespoons white sesame seeds
- 2 large shallots sliced
- ¼ cup extra dry vermouth
- 1 ½ teaspoons kosher salt plus more for the pasta water
- ½ cup raw cashews
- freshly ground black pepper
- 8 ounces whole grain penne or other sturdy shape of pasta

Instructions

1. Preheat your oven to 400°F. Lined a rimmed baking sheet with parchment paper.

2. Place half of the squash pieces on the baking sheet and toss with 1 tablespoon oil and ½ teaspoon of salt.

Roast until the squash is soft and starting to brown, about 10 minutes. Remove from the oven and sprinkle with black and white sesame seeds. Put back in the oven for another 15 minutes, then set aside and keep warm.

3. Meanwhile, heat one tablespoon of the oil in a large pot over low heat. Add the shallots and cook, stirring often, until soft, about 5 minutes. Add the vermouth and bring to a boil, scraping any bits of browned shallots from the bottom of the pot, and cook for another 3 minutes. Transfer the shallots and vermouth to a blender; set aside.

4. Get a pot of salted water boiling for the pasta.

5. Add the remaining raw squash, water, cashews, and remaining teaspoon salt to the pot you cooked the shallots in. The squash should be submerged, so add more water if needed. Bring to a boil. Reduce the heat and simmer gently until you can easily pierce a piece of squash with a fork, about 20 minutes. Let cool slightly, then ladle the vegetables and half the cooking water into the blender with the shallots. Blend on high (being careful to make sure the lid is on tight with a dish towel to cover allowing the steam to escape) until very creamy and smooth, about 2 minutes, using additional water if needed to give it the consistency of a heavy cream. Pour the sauce back into the same saucepan and keep warm over low heat.

6. Add your pasta to the boiling water and cook until al dente (about 1 minute before the specified cooking time on the package). Drain, reserving one cup of the cooking water. Add the pasta to the pot with the sauce and gently stir until the pasta is evenly coated. Add the pasta cooking water by the tablespoonful, if needed, to loosen the sauce.

7. Just before serving, toss the roasted squash and sesame seeds with the pasta. Divide pasta evenly between bowls, drizzle with the rest of the olive oil, and sprinkle with chives. Serve hot.

22. Eggplant Rollatini with Creamy Chard Ricotta

Servings: 6

Ingredients

- 3 medium eggplants
- ½ teaspoon kosher salt plus more for salting the eggplant
- extra virgin olive oil to brush eggplants
- 1 bunch rainbow chard stems separated and diced fine, about 12 leaves
- 2 medium garlic cloves
- 3/4 cup raw cashews soaked water to cover for at least an hour
- 1/2 cup water
- ¼ cup freshly squeezed lemon juice
- freshly ground black pepper
- 1 cup crumbled extra firm tofu
- zest of 1 lemon
- 1/2 teaspoon red pepper flakes
- 2 cups Marinara sauce
- 1 cup Arugula or basil pesto
- Fresh basil to garnish

Instructions

1. Preheat oven to 300°F. Cut the eggplant in half lengthwise and slice into ¼-inch thin slices using a mandolin or a sharp knife. Place the slices on a parchment lined baking sheet and sprinkle with about

1 teaspoon of kosher salt. After 20 minutes, blot dry. Bake for 20 minutes or until soft.

2. Steam the rainbow chard leaves and the garlic cloves for 5 minutes. Place the steamed garlic cloves in a blender and place the leaves on a kitchen towel to dry. Drain the cashews and discard the soaking water. Add the cashews, 1/2 cup fresh water, lemon juice, salt and pepper to the garlic in the blender. Process until creamy, adding more water if needed. Scrape the cashew cream into the bowl.

3. Using a kitchen towel, wring the chard leaves dry. Chop fine and place in a large bowl. Add to the cashew cream.

4. Sauté the chard stems in the oil over medium heat until soft, about 7 minutes. Add to the cashew cream. Add the tofu, lemon zest, and red pepper flakes. Mix well and adjust for salt, pepper and lemon.

5. Fill the bottom of a 9 x 12-inch baking dish with marinara sauce (about 1 ½ cups.) Spoon a heaping tablespoon of ricotta onto the short end of each eggplant slice. Roll up and place in the pan atop the marinara. Repeat until you have about 24 rollatini.

6. Spoon more marinara down the center of the rollatini. Drizzle with pesto and bake for 20 minutes at 375°F.

7. Serve warm, topped with more pesto if needed, and fresh basil sprigs.

23. Whole Grain Penne with Creamy Squash and Sesame

Servings: 4

Ingredients

- 6 cups cubed butternut squash or pumpkin (from 1 large or 2 small squash, about 3 lbs. total), peeled and divided
- 3 tablespoons extra virgin olive oil
- ¼ cup sesame seeds I like to use equal parts white and black.
- 2 tablespoons white sesame seeds
- 2 large shallots sliced
- ¼ cup extra dry vermouth
- 1 ½ teaspoons kosher salt plus more for the pasta water
- ½ cup raw cashews
- freshly ground black pepper
- 8 ounces whole grain penne or other sturdy shape of pasta

Instructions

1. Preheat your oven to 400°F. Lined a rimmed baking sheet with parchment paper.

2. Place half of the squash pieces on the baking sheet and toss with 1 tablespoon oil and ½ teaspoon of salt. Roast until the squash is soft and starting to brown, about 10 minutes. Remove from the oven and sprinkle

with black and white sesame seeds. Put back in the oven for another 15 minutes, then set aside and keep warm.

3. Meanwhile, heat one tablespoon of the oil in a large pot over low heat. Add the shallots and cook, stirring often, until soft, about 5 minutes. Add the vermouth and bring to a boil, scraping any bits of browned shallots from the bottom of the pot, and cook for another 3 minutes. Transfer the shallots and vermouth to a blender; set aside.

4. Get a pot of salted water boiling for the pasta.

5. Add the remaining raw squash, water, cashews, and remaining teaspoon salt to the pot you cooked the shallots in. The squash should be submerged, so add more water if needed. Bring to a boil. Reduce the heat and simmer gently until you can easily pierce a piece of squash with a fork, about 20 minutes. Let cool slightly, then ladle the vegetables and half the cooking water into the blender with the shallots. Blend on high (being careful to make sure the lid is on tight with a dish towel to cover allowing the steam to escape) until very creamy and smooth, about 2 minutes, using additional water if needed to give it the consistency of a heavy cream. Pour the sauce back into the same saucepan and keep warm over low heat.

6. Add your pasta to the boiling water and cook until al dente (about 1 minute before the specified cooking time on the package). Drain, reserving one cup of the

cooking water. Add the pasta to the pot with the sauce and gently stir until the pasta is evenly coated. Add the pasta cooking water by the tablespoonful, if needed, to loosen the sauce.

7. Just before serving, toss the roasted squash and sesame seeds with the pasta. Divide pasta evenly between bowls, drizzle with the rest of the olive oil, and sprinkle with chives. Serve hot.

24. Spicy Salmon Summer Salad

Prep Time: 20 minutes
Cook Time: 10 minutes
Total Time: 30 minutes
Servings: 4

Ingredients

- 1 teaspoon paprika
- 1 teaspoon cumin
- 1/2 teaspoon cayenne pepper
- 1/4 teaspoon coarse sea salt
- 4 4-ounce boneless skin-on salmon filet
- 1 tablespoon extra virgin olive oil

For the salad:

- 4 cups baby greens (arugula,spinach, romaine)
- 1 head Bibb lettuce lightly chopped
- 1 cup fresh or thawed frozen corn
- 2 cups halved grape tomatoes

For the dressing:

- 1/4 cup extra virgin olive oil
- Juice of 1 lime
- 1 tablespoon pure maple syrup

For serving:

- 2 avocados peeled, pitted and sliced
- 2 limes quartered

Instructions

1. In a small bowl, combine the paprika, cumin, cayenne, and salt. Gently rub the spice mixture onto the flesh side of the salmon filets.

2. Heat the oil in a large sauté pan over medium heat. Place the fillets skin-side up in the pan. Cook for 4 minutes, then flip the fillets.

3. Reduce the heat to low, cover, and cook for another 4 to 6 minutes, or until just cooked through.

4. In a medium bowl, combine the spinach, lettuce, corn, and tomatoes. In a small bowl, whisk together all the dressing ingredients. Pour the dressing over the salad and toss.

5. Evenly divide the salad among four plates. Top each with a salmon filet and a few avocado slices. Serve with lime wedges on the side.

25. Cilantro Chutney

Prep Time: 10 minutes

Servings: 0.7 cup

Ingredients

- 1 bunch cilantro stems and leaves washed, dried and roughly chopped (about 1 cup, packed)
- ¼ cup raw unsalted cashews
- 4 tablespoons fresh lemon juice
- 1 teaspoon kosher or sea salt
- 4 teaspoons honey
- ¼ teaspoon ground turmeric
- 1 to 2 small fresh serrano chiles roughly chopped, deseeded for less heat

Instructions

1. Place the cilantro in the bowl of a blender or food processor. Add the rest of the ingredients, except for one of the chiles, and pulse until smooth and pesto-like. Add a few spoonfuls of water to achieve a smooth consistency.

2. Taste; add the last chile if you like it more spicy; add more lemon juice, salt, or honey to taste. It should taste equally fiery, sweet and lemony.

26. Citrusy Salmon Packets with Zoodles and Cilantro Chutney

Prep Time: 15 minutes

Cook Time: 10 minutes

Total Time: 25 minutes

Servings: 4

Ingredients

- 4 4-oz pieces salmon filet skin on, about 1-inch thick
- 1 teaspoon coarse sea salt
- 1/2 cup freshly squeezed orange juice
- 2 tablespoons freshly squeezed lime juice
- 2 tablespoons freshly squeezed lemon juice
- zest of 1 orange
- zest of 1 lemon
- 1 medium butternut squash peeled and bulbous end removed
- 1 zucchini
- 3 tablespoons extra virgin olive oil
- 1 leek white and light green portion thinly sliced
- 2 medium garlic cloves thinly sliced
- 1/4 teaspoon freshly ground black pepper
- 2 blood oranges thinly sliced
- 1 recipe Cilantro Chutney

Instructions

1. Preheat the oven to 400°F.

2. Place the salmon on a rimmed baking dish, skin side down, and sprinkle with a half teaspoon of the salt. In a small bowl, stir together orange juice, lime juice, lemon juice, orange zest, and lemon zest. Pour the juices over the salmon and flip over a few times to coat. Cover the dish and marinate in the fridge for 20 minutes.

3. While the salmon marinates, make the Cilantro Chutney.

4. Place the barrel-shaped part of the butternut squash (the stem end) in the spiralizer. (Save the bulbous, round end for another dish.) Spiralize using the "spaghetti" setting. Place in a bowl. Trim the ends from the zucchini and cut it in half. Spiralize using the same setting. Add to the butternut squash noodles and add 2 tablespoons of the olive oil, the leek, and the garlic. Season with black pepper and an additional pinch of salt.

5. To assemble the packets, lay out 4 15-inch by 24-inch pieces of parchment paper, or one for each serving. Fold each sheet in half, forming a 15 x 12-inch rectangle. Use scissors to cut out a half-moon or heart shape as big as the paper allows. Unfold the half moon of paper, brush half with olive oil, and divide zoodle mixture evenly between each portion. Place fish on top of each noodle mound, skin side down. Layer

blood orange slices over the surface of each salmon filet and drizzle with a few spoonfuls of the marinade.

6. Fold the other half of parchment over and line up the edges. Starting at the top, fold over about ½-inch of the edge, pressing down to make a crisp crease. Continue to work your way around the edge of the packet, making overlapping folds (like pleats), always pressing firmly and creasing the edge so the folds hold. Twist the tip of the heart or moon to finish. If necessary, make a second fold anyplace that doesn't appear tightly sealed.

7. Place packets on a rimmed baking sheet. Cook immediately or refrigerate for later; bringing to room temperature before baking.

8. Bake for 7-8 minutes for medium rare. Cooking time will depend on the thickness of your salmon. Allow a few minutes more if your filets are more than 1-inch thick.

9. To serve, slit open the packets and transfer to a plate or serve in the packets. Top each serving with a generous spoonful of Cilantro Chutney.

27. Pan-Fried Carrots and Asparagus with Dukkah

Prep Time: 10 minutes

Cook Time: 15 minutes

Total Time: 25 minutes

Servings: 4

Ingredients

- 2 bunches slender carrots about 8
- 1 bunch slender asparagus about 10 spears
- 1/2 cup hazelnuts
- 1/2 cup sesame seeds
- 1/4 cup coriander seed
- 3 tablespoons cumin seed
- 1 teaspoon coarse sea salt plus more, to taste
- 1/2 teaspoon freshly ground black pepper
- 3 tablespoons extra virgin olive oil

Instructions

1. Peel or scrub the carrots well. Snap off the bottoms of the asparagus. Place the vegetables on a kitchen towel and blot dry.

2. Preheat the oven to 325°F. Place the hazelnuts on a rimmed baking sheet. Bake for 17 minutes or until

fragrant and darker in color. Transfer to a cutting
board and coarsely chop.

3. Toast the seeds: Place a dry skillet over medium heat.
   Add sesame seeds and twirl gently. When the seeds
   start to pop, they are done. Pour into a small bowl.
   Using the same skillet, toast the cumin seeds over
   medium heat. Remove from the heat as soon as they
   become fragrant and add to the bowl with the sesame
   seeds. Repeat with the coriander seeds, removing
   them from the pan when they start to pop. Using the
   pack of a spoon, slightly crush the seeds. Add
   hazelnuts, salt, and pepper and combine with a spoon.

4. Place a large skillet over medium high heat. When
   hot, add 1 tablespoon of olive oil and warm until it
   starts to shimmer. Add carrots and season with a
   pinch of salt. Sauté over medium heat until brown on
   all sides. Transfer to a plate and set aside.

5. Using the same skillet, add another tablespoon of
   olive oil and warm to a shimmer. Add asparagus and
   season with a pinch of salt. Sauté until brown on all
   sides. Transfer to the plate with the carrots and set
   aside.

6. Warm the last tablespoon of olive oil in the same pan.
   Add 4 tablespoons of dukkah and quickly sauté until
   fragrant. Return carrots and asparagus to the pan and
   toss well until coated with the spice mixture.

28. Pasta Cauliflower Alfredo

Prep Time: 25 minutes

Cook Time: 20 minutes

Total Time: 45 minutes

Servings: 6

Ingredients
- 1 head cauliflower medium-sized
- 1/2 teaspoon kosher or sea salt
- 1 cup raw cashews soaked for at least one hour and drained
- 1 teaspoon truffle salt
- 2 tablespoons nutritional yeast
- 1/4 tsp white pepper
- 1 pound whole grain pasta

Instructions

1. Trim the cauliflower of any discolored leaves. Trim the base of the main stem so that it stands upright. Place the whole head, stem side down, in a pan large enough to contain it when covered. Add water to cover the stem and just the bottom of the cauliflower.

2. Place over high heat, bring to a boil and cover. Reduce the heat to low-medium. Steam for 15 minutes, or until the cauliflower is very soft and a knife or skewer easily pierces through to the core. Steaming times will

vary depending on the size of your cauliflower —
about 13 minutes for small, 15 minutes for medium,
and 18 minutes for a large head.

3. Using tongs or a kitchen towel, transfer the
    cauliflower to a cutting board. Pour the cooking water
    into a measuring cup. Remove the leaves and cut
    them into slivers. Cut the stem from the rest of the
    head, trim off any woody parts, and chop into 2-inch
    pieces. Cut the head of cauliflower into 4 or 5 pieces.

4. Place the steamed cauliflower florets and pieces of
    stem in a blender. Add the cashews, truffle salt,
    nutritional yeast, white pepper and 3/4 cup of the
    cooking water. Blend on medium speed until
    combined, then on high speed until very creamy,
    about 2 minutes. Add more cooking water, if needed,
    to create a pourable, smooth cauliflower cream. Set
    aside.

5. To cook the pasta, bring a large pot of water to a boil.
    Add 1 teaspoon of sea salt and add the pasta. Cook
    until al dente, or still chewy and not quite done. Drain
    over a colander.

6. Pour the cauliflower cream into the same pan used to
    cook the pasta. Warm over medium heat until
    bubbling gently. Add the cooked pasta to the sauce
    and gently combine with a wooden spoon. Once the
    pasta is coated with the alfredo sauce, add the slivered
    cauliflower leaves and warm through.

29. Pumpkin Polenta

Prep Time: 5 minutes

Cook Time: 25 minutes

Total Time: 30 minutes

Servings: 4

Ingredients
- 3 cups almond milk
- 1/4 teaspoon nutmeg
- 3/4 teaspoon kosher salt
- 1/4 teaspoon ground white pepper or black pepper
- 5 tablespoons polenta (such as Bob's Red Mill corn grits not instant)
- 5 tablespoons chickpea flour
- 1 cup pumpkin puree from a can

Instructions

1. Pour the almond milk into a large saucepan and bring to a simmer.

2. Add the nutmeg, salt and pepper.

3. Slowly add the 5 tablespoons of polenta over the simmering milk, whisking continuously. Keep whisking and add the chickpea flour. Cook over very low heat so that the polenta is gently bubbling up,

whisking every few minutes, until the grains are soft, about 10 minutes.

4. Add the pumpkin and whisk until the polenta is smooth and bubbling gently again, about 5 minutes.

5. Using a wooden spoon, vigorously stir the polenta for about 1 minute.

6. Remove the pan from the heat. Taste; adjust for salt and pepper.

30. Shrimp, Tomato, and Chickpea Stew

Prep Time: 35 minutes
Cook Time: 40 minutes
Total Time: 1 hour 15 minutes
Servings: 4-6

Ingredients

- 1/4 cup extra virgin olive oil
- 3 cups cherry tomatoes or 1 14-oz can crushed tomatoes
- 2 teaspoons minced garlic
- 1/2 cup white wine
- 1 pound large shrimp peeled and deveined, about 16-20
- 1 1/2 cups cooked chickpeas cooked from scratch or from one 15-oz. can, see note
- 1/2 teaspoon kosher or sea salt
- freshly ground pepper to taste
- 2 tablespoons fresh chives finely chopped

Instructions

1. Place a large saucepan over medium heat. When the pan is hot, add the olive oil and heat just until it starts to shimmer. Add the cherry tomatoes and the salt, and cook over low-medium heat until the tomatoes start to burst, about 10 minutes.

2. Add the garlic and cook for another 2 minutes, stirring to make sure nothing sticks to the bottom of the pot.

3. Add the white wine and cook for a few minutes to reduce the sauce.

4. Fold in the chickpeas and place the shrimp atop the simmering sauce. Cover the pot and cook over low-medium heat until the shrimp turn pink, about 5 minutes.

5. Taste; adjust the salt and add freshly ground pepper.

6. Just before serving, garnish with chives.

SNACKS

31. Dark Chocolate Granola with Cacao Nibs

Prep Time: 10 minutes

Cook Time: 45 minutes

Total Time: 55 minutes

Servings: 6

Ingredients

- 5 cups old-fashioned rolled oats
- 1 cup sliced almonds
- 2 tablespoons natural cacao powder
- 1 teaspoon cinnamon
- ¾ teaspoon ground cardamom
- 1 cup pure maple syrup
- 2/3 cup extra virgin olive oil
- 1 tsp almond extract
- 1 tsp vanilla extract
- 1 tsp coarse salt
- 1 ounce dark chocolate 70% cacao content or greater
- ½ cup cacao nibs
- Maldon sea salt to taste, optional

Instructions

1. Preheat oven to 350°F and place the rack in the center of the oven. Line a rimmed (18 x 13-inch) baking sheet with parchment paper or a silicon mat.

2. In a large bowl, combine oats, sliced almonds, cacao powder, cinnamon, cardamom, and salt.

3. In a large (4-cup) measuring cup, combine maple syrup, olive oil, almond extract, and vanilla extract using a fork or a whisk.

4. Pour olive oil mixture over the oats and stir to combine. Using a rubber spatula, spread evenly over the baking sheet.

5. Bake for 20 minutes. Rotate baking sheet front to back. Bake another 20 minutes. Pull the pan from the oven and carefully inspect the granola. If it is golden brown throughout and darker brown on the edges, it is done. If not, return to the oven and check it again in 3 minutes. Keep checking until the granola is golden brown but not burning at the edges.

6. Remove from the oven and cool in the pan. Transfer to a large bowl. When the granola is no longer warm, grate the dark chocolate over the bowl using the large holes of a box grater. Stir to evenly distribute the chocolate shards.

7. Add the cacao nibs and stir again.

8. Taste the granola. You may want to add a little more salt to balance the chocolate and bring out its flavor. I like to add a sprinkle of flaky Maldon sea salt. If not, scoop the granola in to an airtight container (I like to use tall Mason jars) and store in a cool place away from sunlight.

9. Enjoy in small portions (less than ¼ cup) as a snack, or sprinkled on berries and yogurt.

32. Lemony Blueberry Chia Seed Tart
Servings: 1

Ingredients

Crust:
- 1/2 cup dates about 6 small or 10 large ones
- 2 cups raw almonds
- 1/4 cup oats
- 1/2 teaspoon kosher or sea salt
- 3 tablespoon extra virgin olive oil
- zest of 1 lemon

Blueberry Chia Seed Jam:
- 2 cups fresh blueberries
- 2 tablespoons pure maple syrup
- 1/4 cup fresh lemon juice
- 2 tablespoons chia seeds

Topping:
- 3 cups fresh blueberries
- Zest of one lemon
- 1 bunch fresh thyme leaves stripped from the stems, plus a few intact sprigs for garnish
- 1 teaspoon coconut palm sugar heaping teaspoon
- Vanilla Bean Cashew Cream optional

Equipment:
- 9 x 9-inch tart pan
- food processor

Instructions

1. Place the dates in a small bowl and cover with water. Soak for 30 minutes. Drain and remove the pits.

2. Preheat the oven to 350°F. Grease the sides and bottom of a 9 x 9-inch tart pan (with a removable bottom) with olive oil.

3. In the bowl of a food processor, place the almonds and pulse until mealy in texture. Add the oats and salt. Pulse a few more times.

4. With the motor running, add one date at a time. Add the olive oil and process until a ball begins to form on the side of the bowl. (If your crust is not balling up, add another spoonful of olive oil.)

5. Press the crust mixture into the prepared tart pan and flatten with the palms of your hands. Press it into the corners and up the sides of the pan to make an even crust. Use the flat side of a glass to press the bottom crust evenly throughout.

6. Bake for 20 minutes, or until the crust is browning on the edges.

7. While the tart shell is baking, make the blueberry chia seed jam. First, zest the lemon and set it aside for the topping. Cut the lemon in half and juice it; you should have about ¼ cup of juice. Put 2 cups of blueberries, 2 tablespoons of maple syrup, and the lemon juice in a small saucepan. Heat to a simmer, stirring occasionally, until the berries burst and release their

juice, about 5 minutes. Stir in the 2 tablespoons of chia seeds and cook over low heat, stirring continuously, until it becomes the consistency of jam. It should start to set up after 1-2 minutes.

8. When the tart shell is done, let it cool for a few minutes. Slather the blueberry chia seed jam over the bottom of the crust in an even layer. Top with half the lemon zest.

9. Arrange the rest of the berries on the surface. Sprinkle with the rest of the lemon zest and the tablespoon of coconut palm sugar.

10. Reduce the oven to 300. Bake the tart for 8-10 minutes, watching carefully to be sure the edges do not burn.

11. Once the tart is completely cool, lift the bottom of the tart pan from the sides. Shower the tart with fresh thyme leaves just before serving, and garnish with a few thyme sprigs. Serve with a dollop of Vanilla Bean Cashew Cream, if using.

33. Rustic Marmalade Cake

Servings: 4

Ingredients

- 1 organic lemon
- 1 organic seedless orange
- 1/2 cup raw almonds
- 1 cup white whole wheat flour
- 1/2 cup almond flour
- 1 tablespoon baking powder
- 4 eggs at room temperature
- 1/2 teaspoon kosher salt
- 1 1/2 cups coconut palm sugar
- 2/3 cup fruity olive oil
- Optional: berries edible blooms, honey Greek yogurt

Instructions

1. Preheat the oven to 325°F.

2. Place the lemon and orange in a saucepan and cover with water. Bring to a boil, reduce heat to medium, and simmer for 30 minutes. Drain and cool the fruit.

3. Spread the almonds on a baking sheet and bake for 10-15 minutes, or until they are toasty brown. When cool, pulse in a food processor until they are the

texture of coarse sand. Remove from the processor and set aside.

4. Increase the oven temperature to 355°F (350°F at sea level).

5. Cut the lemon in half and scoop out and discard the pulp and the seeds. Cut the orange in half.

6. Without cleaning the food processor, add the lemon rind and the whole orange.

7. Pulse until it resembles a thick marmalade.

8. In a small bowl, whisk together the flour, almond flour, and baking powder.

9. Crack the eggs into a mixing bowl and sprinkle with the salt. Using a whisk, beat until foamy, then gradually add the sugar.

10. Fold the white whole wheat and almonds flours into the egg and sugar mixture. Add the "marmalade," almonds, and the olive oil. Stir with a wooden spoon until a thick batter forms.

11. Grease the springform pan with a few teaspoons of olive oil. Scrape the batter into the pan and smooth over the top.

12. Bake for about an hour, or until a toothpick placed in the center of the cake comes out clean.

13. Once cool, release from the pan and garnish with fresh berries, edible blooms,or a dollop of honey Greek yogurt.

34. Cacao Tahini Date Balls

Prep Time: 20 minutes

Servings: 12

Ingredients

- 10 Medjool dates pits removed
- 1 1/2 cups hazelnut flour
- 1/3 cup tahini
- 1 teaspoon cinnamon
- 1/4 teaspoon cardamom
- 2 tablespoons cacao powder
- 2 teaspoons water
- 1/2 teaspoon sea salt
- 1 cup sunflower seeds
- 1/4 cup sesame seed

Instructions

1. Put all ingredients except the sesame seeds in the bowl of a food processor. Pulse until the dough becomes sticky and pinches easily together, adding more water if necessary.

2. Place the sesame seeds on a pie plate or rimmed baking sheet.

3. Scoop out 2 tablespoons of the dough and roll into a ball with your hands. Compress to make sure the dough holds together.

4. Roll in sesame seeds.

5. Store in an airtight container in the fridge. The date
    balls will keep for up to 5 days.

35. Za'atar Spiced Pecans

Prep Time: 10 minutes
Cook Time: 15 minutes
Total Time: 25 minutes
Servings: 6

Ingredients

- 1/2 cup white sesame seeds
- 1/2 cup oregano
- 4 tbsp sumac
- 1 1/2 cups raw pecans
- 3 tbsp extra virgin olive oil
- 1/2 tsp coarse sea salt such as flaky Maldon salt

Instructions

1. Preheat the oven to 375°F.

2. Make the za'atar: In a small bowl, stir together the sesame seeds, sumac, and oregano. You will have more za'atar than needed for this recipe. (See notes for other ways to use it.)

3. In a small bowl, toss pecans with olive oil, 1 tablespoon za'atar, and the salt.

4. Pour the spiced pecans onto a large rimmed baking sheet lined with parchment paper. Spread out so they are all in contact with the baking sheet.

5. Roast in the oven for about 15 minutes. Check on them at 12 minutes and keep checking every few minutes until toasty brown.

6. Remove from the oven and cool. Lift up each side of the parchment paper to create a scoop to pour them into a jar with a tight-fitting lid. Serve warm as an appetizer. Sprinkle over salads. And, of course, these Za'atar Spiced Pecans are perfect for snacking. They'll stay fresh for up to 1 month.

36. Almond Butter Baked Apples

Prep Time: 10 minutes
Cook Time: 40 minutes
Total Time: 50 minutes
Servings: 4

Ingredients

- 4 apples medium-sized
- 1/2 cup almond butter or peanut, cashew or other nut or seed butter
- 1 date pit removed, finely chopped
- 1 tablespoon crystallized ginger finely chopped
- 1 tablespoon extra virgin olive oil
- 1 tablespoon pure maple syrup
- 1/4 cup cashews raw or roasted and salted
- 1/2 teaspoon cinnamon
- 4 tablespoons Vanilla Bean Cashew Cream or unsweetened Greek yogurt

Instructions

1. Preheat oven to 400°F.

2. Wash the apples and blot dry. Using a vegetable peeler or apple corer, remove the core and stem end of the apple, making sure not to puncture all the way through the bottom of the apple.

3. Stuff each apple with a spoonful of almond butter.

4. Sprinkle the chopped dates and crystalized ginger over the apples.

5. Once each apple is packed and a little overflowing with stuffings, snuggle into a rimmed baking dish. Stir olive oil and maple syrup together in a small cup and pour over the apples.

6. Bake for 35 to 40 minutes, or until the apples are tender and a pool of juices collects in the bottom of the baking dish. Baking time will depend on the size of your apples, so check them after 30 minutes and probe with a cake tester or skewer. If it easily slides through the apple, they are done.

7. To serve, dollop each apple with a generous spoonful of Vanilla Bean Cashew Cream. Sprinkle with cinnamon and top with cashews.

37. Tahini-Swirled Brownie Bites
Servings: 6

Ingredient

- ¼ cup extra virgin olive oil plus more for greasing the pan
- 2 large eggs at room temperature
- ½ cup pure maple syrup
- ⅓ cup no-sugar-added applesauce
- 1 teaspoon vanilla extract
- ¾ cup almond flour
- ½ cup natural cocoa powder not Dutch-processed
- ½ teaspoon kosher salt
- ½ cup 60% or greater dark chocolate (3 ounces) chopped
- ⅓ cup tahini well-stirred and at room temperature

Instructions

1. Preheat your oven to 400°F. Line an 8-by-8-inch pan with parchment paper and grease the sides with olive oil.

2. Whisk the eggs, maple syrup, applesauce, oil, and vanilla in a large bowl until combined. Fold in the almond flour, cocoa powder, and salt until few streaks remain. Fold in the chopped chocolate until evenly distributed.

3. Pour the batter into the prepared pan and smooth the top with a spoon. Dollop the tahini evenly over the batter in about 9 places. Use a skewer or a knife to swirl them throughout to create a marbled effect.

4. Bake for 25 minutes or until the edges are set and the center is only slightly wobbly. For best results, cool completely and chill in the pan for at least 30 minutes (or freeze for 15 minutes) before cutting. Invert the brownies from the pan onto a cutting board, flip over, and cut into 1-inch squares.

38. A Better-For-You Chocolate Chunk Cookie

Servings: 32 cookies

Ingredients

- ¾ cup chickpea flour
- ¾ cup buckwheat flour
- 1 teaspoon baking powder
- ½ teaspoon baking soda
- ¼ cup natural cacao powder
- ¾ kosher salt
- ¾ cup coconut palm sugar
- ½ cup extra virgin olive oil
- 1 large egg
- 1 teaspoon pure vanilla extract
- 2 teaspoons water
- 6 ounces chopped bittersweet chocolate, 60-70% cacao about 1 cup
- Pinches Maldon salt or other flaky salt

Instructions

1. In a large bowl, whisk together the chickpea and buckwheat flours, baking powder, baking soda, cocoa powder, and salt; set aside.

2. Combine the sugar and olive oil in the bowl of an electric mixer. Beat on medium speed until combined. Add the egg and vanilla and beat again until smooth. Scrape down the sides with a rubber spatula.

3. Add the dry ingredients and beat on low speed until combined, about 2 minutes. Scrape down the sides again.

4. Separate about 2 tablespoons of the larger pieces of chocolate to press into the tops of the cookies before baking. On low speed, fold in the rest of the chocolate, then scrape down the sides and mix until evenly incorporated.

5. Using a tablespoon measure, scoop out the cookie dough, roll into a ball, and place on the prepared baking sheets, leaving 1 inch between cookies. Press a chocolate piece onto the top of each cookie. Refrigerate for at least 1 hour and up to overnight, tightly covered with plastic wrap.

6. Thirty minutes before baking, preheat the oven to 350°F. Line two rimmed baking sheets with parchment paper.

7. Bake for 11 to 13 minutes, or until the edges are set. The center of the cookies will still be soft but will finish cooking as they cool. Sprinkle the top of each cookie with a pinch of flaky salt.

8. Let the cookies cool for at least 15 minutes before serving. (This allows them to finish cooking.)

39. Spiced Nuts with Turmeric and Garam Masala

Servings: 3 cup

Ingredients

- 3 cups mixed unsalted raw nuts (I like equal parts cashews walnuts, and almonds)
- 3 tablespoons avocado or extra virgin olive oil
- 2 teaspoons garam masala see note below
- 1 teaspoon kosher salt
- 1 teaspoon ground chile powder
- 1 teaspoon coconut palm sugar
- 1 teaspoon ground turmeric
- 1 tablespoon chickpea flour

Instructions

1. Preheat your oven to 350°F. Line a rimmed baking sheet with parchment paper; set aside.

2. Combine the nuts and oil in a large mixing bowl and toss until evenly coated. Add the remaining ingredients and toss well so that each nut is evenly coated. Transfer to the prepared baking sheet and smooth into an even layer.

3. Bake until the nuts are fragrant and lightly toasted, about 30 minutes. Check the nuts after 15 minutes, give them a toss, and assess how fast they are cooking. If your oven runs hot, they may be done.

4. Serve warm, or cool completely and save in an airtight
   container for up to 2 weeks.

40. Pumpkin Blueberry Muffins

Prep Time: 10 minutes

Cook Time: 40 minutes

Total Time: 50 minutes

Servings: 12

Ingredients

- 1 cup oat flour
- 1 cup almond flour
- ¼ cup hemp seeds (also called hemp hearts) plus 1 tablespoon to top the muffins
- 2 teaspoons baking powder
- 1 tablespoon ground flaxseeds
- 1 teaspoon ground cinnamon
- ½ teaspoon kosher salt
- 1 cup pumpkin puree from a can
- ⅔ cup coconut palm sugar
- ½ cup extra virgin olive oil
- 1 teaspoon pure vanilla extract
- 1 teaspoon almond extract
- 2 large eggs
- 2 cups blueberries fresh or frozen

Instructions

1. Preheat your oven to 350°F. Line a 12-cup muffin tin with paper liners and set aside.

2. In a large bowl, whisk together the oat and almond flours, ¼ cup of the hemp hearts, the baking powder, ground flaxseed, cinnamon, and ½ teaspoon salt; set aside.

3. In a separate large bowl, whisk together the pumpkin, sugar, olive oil, vanilla, and almond extracts. Whisk in the eggs one at a time. Fold the dry ingredients into the wet ones until just combined.

4. Gently fold 1⅓ cups of the blueberries into the muffin batter. Divide the batter evenly between the muffin cups.

5. Divide the remaining ⅔ cup blueberries over the tops of the muffins and gently press them into the batter. Sprinkle with the additional tablespoon of hemp hearts.

6. Bake for 38 to 42 minutes for standard muffins, or until a cake tester or small wooden skewer inserted into muffins comes out clean. For mini muffins, check for doneness starting at 32 minutes.

7. These muffins are best the day they are made or the next day. Warm day-old muffins in the oven at 300°F for 10 minutes. To freeze, wrap in plastic wrap and store in the freezer for up to 6 months.